A
Higher
Calling

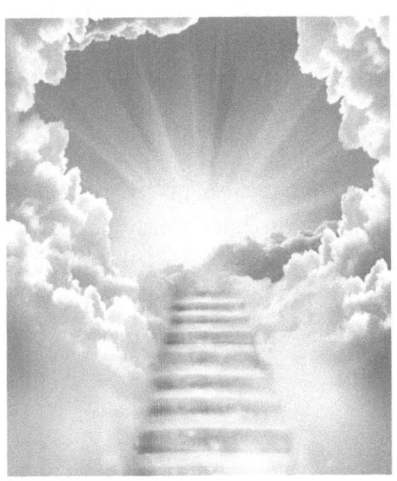

Sharon Lynn Menzel

Library of Congress Control Number:		2011916676
ISBN:	Hardcover	978-1-4653-6798-3
	Softcover	978-1-4653-6797-6
	Ebook	978-1-4653-6799-0

To order additional copies of this book, contact:
Xlibris Corporation
1-888-795-4274
www.Xlibris.com
Orders@Xlibris.com
105176

Contents

Introduction

have been contemplating for years writing a book. I wasn't ready to sit down and do it. I finally decided that now is the time to write it. For years, people have been telling me to write a book about my life. At face value, one would not think that my life would be any different than anyone else's. I have pondered this exact question for years. I take every day as a new day, a new challenge, and a new adventure. Life has not been easy for me, but I believe that I have a knack for turning lemons into lemonade. It wasn't until the last two years that I think I finally got it. I have watched the signs, ignored the signs actually, and I am finally coming to grips with the fact that this book is the next step in my journey. Writing this book is somewhat of a cleansing for me, and I hope that you too may find solace within its pages.

This book is dedicated to my daughter, Kara, for without her, life would have no meaning for me. In addition, this book is dedicated to all my friends and family that have nudged me when I needed nudging and given me a tongue-lashing in my moments of weakness.

I would be remiss to not tell you my life story as this is what shapes my very existence. It is a difficult one to tell and full of many unbelievable stories. This is why everyone always told me to write a book. I have come to grips with the fact that I may not live very long, and it has made me stronger. I want to experience everything possible. I hope that within these pages you will find solace. It always seems that someone has it worse than I do. I never really considered that my life was bad or difficult. I hope as well that this book might give you the inspiration to pick yourself up and dust yourself off if that is the point in your life that you are at. Everyone kept telling me to write a book. So I have written it now. I don't think that God is done with me even yet. We shall see. What a wonderful thing it is to be alive and be able to write this book. My goal in writing this book is to let people know that no matter how bad things get, there is always hope! I have beaten all the odds, and you can too!

Chapter 1

The Beginning

I was born in West Palm Beach, Florida, on December 15, 1966, at 4:20 PM to Ronald and Sandra Shetron. I have one sister, Beth, and one brother, Ronnie (or Sage, as he likes to be called).

I don't remember much about the first few years of my life. I was plagued with migraine headaches since age five. I had a very turbulent childhood. My grandfather on my father's side was a very stern man. He was the love of my life. My parents struggled with the typical challenges of parenting. We were raised under the premise that children should be seen and not heard and "Spare the rod, spoil the child."

Department of Children and Families was called to my home multiple times as a child for what we used to call corporal punishment.

Many things can be said for corporal punishment. I am not a believer in corporal punishment. My daughter is twenty-three years old and has never been struck one time in her life. I believe that my upbringing taught me values, morals, and ethics. It made me a very strong person. Although I do not believe that beating the tar out of your children is effective, I survived, and we will leave it at that.

My health issues started at age five with the headaches. At age seven, I was skating at a skating rink and fell. I could not stand up. I was rushed to the hospital, and they found that I had a distal femur bone tumor in my left leg. They told my parents that I would never walk again. They told them that the tumor was right by the growing space and that my leg would probably not grow any further. Well, I narrowly escaped that plight as I can walk, and my leg is only about a half an inch shorter than the other one.

As a child, I was very timid and scared. I had many childhood traumas, which I will not go into in this book.

I had newspaper routes from age nine. My mother would drive me on my paper routes when it rained and if she was home early. When I was twelve, she drove me on my afternoon paper route, and when I leaned out the door to throw the paper out the van, she cut to the other side of the street. I fell out of the side door of the van and cracked an iron drain grate and concrete curb with my head. Everything was blurry and spinning. The elderly people on my paper route came running out to help. My mother put me in the van and took me home. Hours later, I woke up vomiting and with a violent headache. My mother finally took me to the ER in the early morning hours. I had a blood clot behind my eardrum and five basal skull fractures. I spent several days in the hospital.

We were sent to private schools through middle school. My parents provided a concrete foundation for our education. I had a love of music and reading. I started playing the piano at six years old. I took two years of lessons and was pretty much self-taught after that. I picked up many more instruments along the way. I currently play eleven instruments.

I always struggled with math from the time that I cracked my head. I have an above-average IQ. I was very bright and very self-driven. I wanted very badly to graduate from high school and leave home. I wanted to go to college, and I wanted to be a doctor.

When I was sixteen, my uncle Bob, whom I was very close to, died of pancreatic cancer. I wanted to find a cure for pancreatic cancer. After I graduated from high school, I wanted to go on to college. We were not a wealthy family and made ends meet where we could. We grew up with very few personal belongings and toys. We did not have anything extra. I always seemed to be hungry and wanting for something in my life that I never could put my finger on.

After I graduated from high school, I asked my dad to send me to college. He said he could not afford to send me to college and to find my own way. I promptly went down to see the air force recruiter and enlisted in the US Air Force. The air force was the best thing that ever happened to me despite the trials and tribulations I endured.

The Air Force

I went into the air force in 1985, after completing high school. I went to basic training at Lackland Air Force Base in 1985. I was first stationed at England Air Force Base, Louisiana. There I met my husband, David Thomas Menzel. I was originally enlisted as a recreation specialist. I was a woman in a man's job. I worked in the sports-and-fitness facility. I had issues with racially discriminating men. I filed a complaint with the squadron commander. The men in the sports-and-fitness facility did not want a woman working in the facility.

I was transferred to the recreation area shortly after I filed the complaint. I was given a job twenty-two miles from the base at Lake Cotile. I worked with many retirees and had a wonderful career for the next few years. I earned my rank quickly, being an E-5 in four years.

I had cross-trained into Personnel. I was given a job as a customer service representative and worked in many facets of Personnel for the remainder of my career.

I got married in November of 1987 and got pregnant right away. I had been battling migraine headaches, and the military put me on hormone blockers to keep the headaches under control. I weighed all of 110 pounds, and my clothes became very tight in the waist two months after I knew I got pregnant. I didn't use birth control, and I knew as soon as I got pregnant.

The military told me that I had a negative HCG test and I tried multiple times to explain to them that they had me on hormone blockers and they wouldn't get a positive test. I finally convinced a doctor that there was something wrong, and he ordered a CAT scan.

The military doctor determined that I had a ten-pound tumor, and they were going to cut it out that weekend. I refused to let them cut me until they got a better test. At that time, the ultrasound machine was broken. They finally did the ultrasound on the following Monday and decided that I was pregnant. They based my due date on forty-four weeks from that date. However, I had been pregnant already for two months.

Time passed quickly, and I kept going into labor. They would stop my labor and say it wasn't time. My due date was the end of November, according to the doctor. I started going into labor in September, which would have been the right time to deliver. They did not deliver my daughter until November, and my water had been slowly dripping out for a month and a half. Finally, she was in enough fetal distress that they had to take her C-section.

The doctor who delivered her was a contractor, and he smelled of alcohol when he came in. I asked for another doctor, and they refused. He ripped me open and took her out. She was so burnt that you could roll twenty-two-inch pieces of skin off her body. She peeled from head to toe.

She was born Kara Alyssa Menzel on November 22, 1988. Thirteen months later, I was still bleeding from having my daughter. I had strange-looking discharge coming out of me. I went to the man who delivered me, and he said that I was fine. I told him that I was going downtown to a civilian doctor. He and the hospital commander told me that if I went downtown, I would be prosecuted to the fullest extent of the law. I told him I really didn't care, but I was going.

I went downtown to a civilian gyn doctor. He diagnosed me with a retained placenta. I asked if he would write me a letter, and he did. I returned to the base to a new gyn doctor and showed him the letter. He told me that this was not possible. He eventually scheduled me for surgery fourteen months after my daughter was born to have the placenta removed. The military called it a Dillation and Curettage.

My daughter began having health problems right away. By age two, I had convinced my military flight surgeon that there was something wrong with her. I called St. Jude's and spoke with Dr. Herrod about Kara. He told me to have the flight surgeon draw a certain blood test, inoculate her with three injections, and then draw blood again thirty days later. He wanted it frozen and sent to St. Jude's.

I received a phone call the day after I had the blood sent to St. Judes that Kara had hypogammaglobulinemia. Kara was diagnosed terminally ill at age two. The way the doctors explained it was that she would have to have gamma globulin infusions each month in order to hopefully stay alive. I was told that she had limited to no IgG levels in her blood.

I drove back and forth to Memphis, Tennessee, to St. Jude's every month to get Kara's blood infusions to keep her healthy.

With budget cuts, the government closed England Air Force Base in 1992, and we were transferred to Homestead Air Force Base. We moved into Homestead Air Force Base with a twenty-five-foot and twenty-eight-foot U-Haul on July 3, 1992.

On August 28, 1992, Hurricane Andrew blew through Homestead, Florida. We had a five-bedroom, four-bath house that was two stories. Andrew took the top floor off the house and caved in most parts of the bottom floor. We lost everything that we ever had. I stood out on the tarmac at the base, out processing three thousand-plus people off the base. We lost everything that we had ever owned in that hurricane.

In the military, you have a special code that is on your file called a Q code when you have a family member with health issues. The code on our file was because of Kara and made it so that the military could not transfer us to any base that could not handle Kara's medical care.

Due to the code, the colonel at Personnel for the air force told me to take off and check out the areas around the bases in Florida and Georgia to see if they could handle Kara's care.

My sister and I drove to Eglin Air Force Base, but there was no housing available because many of the hurricane victims were being reassigned there. My husband was a jet engine mechanic, so we had to stay at bases that used airplanes he was trained to work on. We ended up at Moody Air Force Base, Georgia, because we could use Shands Hospital for Kara's care.

We settled into our new assignment in Valdosta, Georgia. I drove Kara to Shands each month for infusions. Finally after a few months, the doctor suggested that we put a central-line port into her chest, which would allow us to do infusions at home instead of coming to the hospital each month. We agreed and had the port placed. My squadron commander as well as his wife became very close to Kara. Kara became very attached and always wanted his wife around for infusions. She also went to the doctors with us as well. Soon, it became too much as Kara wanted her around all the time. I asked the commander to please tell his wife to back off. He told me that unless a psychiatrist told him to have his wife back off, he would not. I explained that it was detrimental to Kara.

In May of 1993, I took my daughter's medical records, and I went to see a psychiatrist. I told my commander that I had an appointment after work to see the psychiatrist. The psychiatrist wrote me a letter for my commander that said that he needed to tell his wife to back off for the health of my daughter.

While I was at the psychiatrist, my commander beeped me and ordered me to return to base. It was six thirty at night. I did as instructed and returned to base. My commander met me at the squadron where he had a base psychiatrist with him. He and the first sergeant ordered me to go to the base hospital with them. I explained to my commander that I had the letter from the psychiatrist. He would not even look at the letter or her medical records.

When I got to the hospital, they said that they were admitting me to South Georgia Medical Center for an evaluation. No one ever told me what exactly they thought was wrong. I was placed in the psychiatric unit at South Georgia Medical Center for the night. I was told that I would see a team of doctors in the morning and they would determine what to do with me.

The next morning, I met with three psychiatrists. I showed them my daughter's medical records and the letter from the downtown civilian psychiatrist. The doctors said that I suffered from stress and had extenuating circumstances because my daughter was terminally ill. The doctors recommended that they put me on leave for a couple of weeks and that the commander should butt out of my life. The commander decided that this was not going to happen and ordered that I be transported to Eglin Air Force Base, Florida, to be placed in the psychiatric unit. He said that I suffered from factitious disorder by proxy. This means that I was making up what was wrong with my daughter for attention.

I was transported by ambulance four hours to Eglin Air Force Base. I met with the psychiatrist and showed him Kara's records. He would not even look at them. He told me I made it up. I tried everything to get out. I met with the chaplain multiple times. I finally called my congressman. A lieutenant colonel nurse finally looked at Kara's records, and she believed me. She was instrumental in getting me released six weeks after I was admitted. I would never have gotten out because they wanted me to admit that I was lying. I said, "How can I be lying when I have these records right here?"

My colonel had wanted to have my daughter around more, and with me locked up, they were seeing her all the time.

I finally was released from the psychiatric unit in late June. I went immediately back to base and put together a discharge package based on the fact that I had a terminally ill child. My commander refused to sign it. I went to the base commander, wing commander, and hospital commander, and my package was finally signed. I had military documents that supported my case. I kept asking why they thought I had a Q code if my daughter was not sick. I was stationed at Moody Air Force Base because of the Q code. It didn't matter.

I took leave for the next three weeks and went home to Florida and found a job. I returned to the base on my last day in the military, July 7, 1993, to out process. I was being honorably discharged on a hardship based on the fact that I had a terminally ill child. My package was approved by air force headquarters in Texas. So I guess you would ask yourself how I was discharged for the same reason that I was locked away. They said that I made it up but then approved my discharge package for having a terminally ill child.

I went home, packed my clothes, and moved to Florida. I left Kara with Dave for a few weeks until I got settled, and then I went back to Georgia and took Kara and her clothes.

During my days in the military, there were many wonderful times and many learning experiences. I was in temporary duty in Norwich, England, at RAF Sculthorpe. On August 2, 1990, we were scheduled to come home, and Desert Shield kicked off. In the military, when both parents are on active duty, you must have a dependent care folder, which designates who gets your child if you both go to war. In our case, it was my mother. I was in England trying to make arrangements for my mom to come get Kara because Dave was heading to Saudi as well. Unfortunately, his father was diagnosed with cancer, and they let him stay home.

The military is a wonderful establishment that taught me many important life lessons. One major takeaway for me was that things are not always going to be good or under your control. You must stay strong and fight for what is right. I spent many years of my life fighting for what was right. I was in the military through Desert Shield and Storm and gained many life experiences. I was part of the Twenty-Third Tactical Fighter Wing and the Seventy-Fifth Tactical Fighter Squadron. We were the Flying Tigers. We flew the A-10s that flew air-to-ground missions. We had the tiger's teeth on the nose of our planes.

The military is very frustrating at times as well. Before I separated, it took the signature of a full-bird colonel to get an ink pen, yet pilots were flying cross-country missions to Maine to bring lobsters back for parties. There were a significant amount of disparities between the enlisted and officer ranks in the military. I guess it is that way in civilian life as well. We chalk it up to learning experiences. I would do it all over again. For me, it made me feel as though I was a part of something important. I was proud to wear the uniform and to be a part of history.

Chapter 3

Starting Over

*L*ife had become very difficult for me once I got out of the air force. Dave stayed in the air force and was in Georgia, and I had Kara by myself in Florida. I worked full-time and went to school at night to better myself. I had to take her to the doctors all the time, and she was about to start kindergarten. She still had monthly blood infusions.

Kara was very intelligent and had many talents from a young age. I decided when I was younger that I never wanted to raise my child the way I was raised. No reflection on my parents; I just wanted better for my daughter. College was important to me because I would have been a doctor had I had the ability to go to college and not join the air force. My parents did the best they could, but I was determined to do better. Everything that I did and all the extra hours at work were going to mean for me that my daughter would have a great childhood. My goal was to raise her with no childhood trauma. I am happy to report that other than the many battles with her medical, I succeeded. I wanted to make sure that I pursued every talent she had, within reason.

Kara started playing soccer at age four. I coached every team she was ever on until she joined travel teams. She attended educational summer camps every summer, as well as the sports camps. Kara was an avid soccer player, and that kept us on the field every day.

In middle school, she got into trouble and started running track to avoid being grounded. My daughter with no immune system had always been very active. In fact, she had a home nurse, Trish, that would come for years each month and do her blood infusions at home. She would hang her IV bag on a hanger and let her go out and climb her favorite tree. It is amazing how people touch your lives and make things okay with something as simple as hanging an IV bag on a hanger. Blood infusions took eight hours each time and were performed once per month.

Kara ran all through high school becoming district and regional champion as well as many state and all-county, all-conference titles. She even started pole vaulting, to my dismay. I was determined that this child would be dead from her antics if her health didn't kill her.

I sent her to Italy and Greece her junior year of high school and Japan on her senior year. She had learned Chinese and Spanish in school and took Japanese in college.

Once she got into high school, I went back to school once again to finish my degree. I finally received my associate's degree in 1998. I went on to receive my bachelor's degree in 2005 and my MBA in 2007.

My daughter attended private Catholic school. I worked as an office manager then recruiter and eventually on to a human resource director. I had a consulting business, so I had the time to give the attention to Kara that she needed. I traveled significantly. I was very fortunate to have my best friend at home, who helped take care of Kara. She took her to school every day and ran around with her for me.

Chapter 4

The Battles

Kara attended St. Mark Catholic School since first grade. In fourth grade, she was visiting her father, and a lady took a swing at her head for letting a boat loose at a fishing camp. Kara had never been struck before, and as soon as Dave dropped her off, she started sneezing. She had been hospitalized on and off most her life. She developed epilepsy at age five. She was eleven that time, and as soon as she saw me, she started sneezing. She sneezed around the clock every second for sixty-one days. I finally took her to an acupuncturist and a hypnotist.

We found out what happened, and she slowly stopped sneezing. She had been hospitalized four different times and was being fed through a PIC line in her arm. Kara was sixty pounds until tenth grade in high school. She lost twenty pounds, and they wanted me to take her to India where they did a procedure called a transnasal vidian neurectomy. I politely refused and said that we would figure it out. She missed nine weeks of school. Thank the Lord her godmother was a teacher there, and she gave her tests and proctored her homework. They would not let her come to school because she was disruptive.

When Kara was in fourth grade, the day before spring break, I received a call from the Department of Children and Families. They stated that they received a call that Kara was being abused. They came to the house with a police officer. The poor police officer apologized profusely for being there and stated that there was no way this was an abused child. However, they had to do their job. I was being accused of Munchausen syndrome. I told the DCF worker that there is no way that I could give Kara what she has. I would have had to remove all her blood, remove the gamma globulin, and then put it back in. I asked the worker where she saw a billion-dollar lab. After nine months, I was cleared of all charges.

Many years later, I went to work for DCF, and as I had suspected, the principal of the school had turned us in, saying that Kara was not in school. The principal had it in for us and wanted Kara out of the school. However, it is difficult to throw out a straight-A student that gives you no trouble. It was a war between the principal and me after that.

When Kara was in fifth grade, she started coming home with strange injuries. Kara was always different because she spent many years in hospitals and was very ill. After the third head injury and a back injury, I went to the school. The principal said she was fine and they were just freak accidents. Kara would not tell me what happened exactly. She would say she accidently got shoved into a concrete wall or pushed down the stairs. This continued and became progressively worse. I kept going into school about it.

When Kara was in seventh grade, the same children shoved her into the concrete wall in the gym. Kara fled the gym because there was no teacher. She hid in the bathroom. Her friend came and got her out. When class was out, she was heading up the stairs, and the kids threw her backpack up the stairs out on an overhang and shoved her into the wall on the stairs. Kara ran and hid in her locker. The fifth grade teacher saw her hide and went and got her. I received a phone call from a parent that my daughter had been hurt. I immediately went to the school and asked Kara what had happened. She told me who hurt her. I went to the principal and gave her the names of the kids that had done it. She started by telling me that she would do all she could to correct the situation and then implied that maybe my daughter needed to be homeschooled because she really didn't fit in. I told her it didn't matter that she was not like every kid but that she needed to be protected. This was a private school, and there was no reason for the bullying that was occurring. The principal finally looked at me and said that there was going to be a meeting the following day between herself and Kara's teachers and that my husband and I would need to be there.

Dave and I both went in and sat down in front of all of Kara's teachers. No teacher would say a word. The principal started by saying that Kara was a discipline problem. I asked her in the eight years that Kara had been there, how many times did she receive a check mark. The principal replied she didn't know. I told her that I could tell her that Kara had received four check marks in school in eight years. I knew this because every time she got one, she came home crying. You received a check mark for any violation: talking, being out of line, uniforms, etc.

I then asked what the next step was for a discipline-problem child, and she said that they sent a note home. I asked how many of these she had, and the principal replied none. I asked what was next, and she said that they would receive detention. I asked how many times in eight years Kara had detention. She replied none. I told her that I failed to see a discipline problem and that this was a witch hunt. The principal then handed me a letter that she wanted me to open. I told her that I did not think it was appropriate for me to open it in front of everyone because I pretty much could figure out what it said.

To my surprise, I was wrong in thinking it was a warning letter. The letter stated that she was a danger to the school because she fled a classroom and that she needed inpatient psychiatric care before she could return to school. I asked the principal how long she considered inpatient care to be before returning. The principal told me a few months. I politely excused myself and my husband and went and enrolled my daughter in public school. I did file a lawsuit against the diocese of Palm Beach, and it received newspaper and television time for her story. I dropped the suit years later because it was not worth disrupting everyone's lives.

During all these trials and tribulations, my mother had been diagnosed with liver cancer and given sixty days to live. It was a very trying time as my brother and sister and I lived at a hospice with my mother. We did everything for her the last six weeks she was alive. I never was close to my mom, but let me tell you what a humbling experience it is to be holding someone's hand when they pass. She was very distraught and didn't really know what was going on. I was very fortunate that I could make peace with her before she passed.

Before she died, she made me swear that I would go to the Mayo Clinic for my headaches. I promised that I would. My mother passed in 2000. Thank God for my sister and her husband, who took care of my mom and moved my mom and dad in with them. My mother was a lot of work.

Dave came home on leave in June of 2001. He was working in the yard with us and crashed out for the night. My father had a heart attack and was in ICU. On June 19, 2001, I got up and went to the hospital. Dave had orders to Hill Air Force Base, Utah. He was supposed to go get the U-Haul and load up while I was at the hospital. He was drunk that morning and put Kara in the car with him to go get the U-Haul. He had a massive stroke while driving down a major highway in West Palm Beach.

I had just walked into the house, and I got a call on my cell phone from a lady who said that she had Kara. She explained that my husband had a heart attack while driving, and Kara crashed the car into a pole to get him out. The police department received five calls that day. It was a combination of pedestrian versus motorcycle and pedestrians versus car. The pole came down on Kara's side of the car, and she flattened herself out. She climbed over her dad and ran for help. She was twelve years old.

My sister and I spent the next six months living in Tampa in an effort to rehabilitate Dave. I lived in a hotel and pushed him to and from therapy each day. They said if he lived, he would be a vegetable. He is paralyzed on the right, and he suffers from severe aphasia, but he is alive and well. He did develop horrible grand mal seizures from the stroke but is doing okay.

I once had a veterans administration doctor stop doing an MRI on him and asked me what happened to him. I explained that he had a stroke, and the doctor said that he had patients with better-looking brains that lived in the hospital full time. Dave only has 3 percent of his brain alive, but he functions well.

Life for the next few years was very challenging with taking care of Dave and keeping Kara going. He was in the hospital at least once a year with grand mal Seizures. Both of his parents and his brother died all through those few years.

Chapter 5

The Epic Battle

About the same time, I started suffering from severe kidney stones and blood in my urine. The doctors kept telling me that I was fine. I had been diagnosed with pseudotumor cerebri by the Mayo Clinic. This is a condition where the cranial pressure in your head is above normal. Normal cranial pressure is 115. My pressure on a spinal tap was over 500.

They put me on a drug called Diamox that was supposed to keep the pressure down. Unfortunately, it didn't work and started my bout with kidney stones. I was off the drug, and the kidney stones worsened. I would be fine and then get horrific pain in my side. This went on and on. No doctor ever did a dye test on my kidneys.

I moved to Cape Canaveral because Kara had been invited to run with Holy Trinity Episcopal. The day before Thanksgiving in 2007, I woke up to having purple urine. The doctor ordered a dye test on my kidney, and it was found that I had a small cyst in the pelvis of the kidney. I went to see the urologist, and he said that we can watch it or go see what it was. I opted to see what it was. My mother had died from cancer, and I wanted to make sure it was not cancer.

I have had problems with tumors growing over the years. They went in on December 15, 2007, and did a biopsy. It turned out to be renal cell carcinoma. They removed my first kidney, ureter, and a piece of my bladder in January 2008. I went on chemotherapy for the cancer and hoped it would stop. Instead, it continued to spread to the bladder. I had eight bladder tumors removed over the next few months. I was being followed by Mayo, Cleveland Clinic, and the urologist in Cape Canaveral.

I went to Cleveland Clinic in Ohio in September 2009, and they checked the kidney and said it was clean. I had suffered from multiple cancer tumors on the bladder and remaining ureter. The cancer was now transitional cell carcinoma and papillary urothelial carcinoma. It continued to spread, and they kept cutting pieces out and putting me on chemo. I went through BCG chemo and mitomycin-C chemo. Nothing stopped the cancer.

In January 2010, the Mayo Clinic found a tumor on the top of my bladder around the ureter. It had gotten out of the ureter.

They also found that my good kidney was 60 percent covered in cancer. There was no way around losing my second kidney unless I wanted to die. Wanting to die I did. I figured I had endured so much and there was no way that I could live without the second kidney.

My daughter and I had spent part of the summer touring Europe. We climbed mountains and everything, and I had one kidney. I was back at work eight days after losing the first kidney. My sister took fantastic care of me, and I recovered quickly. I prayed and prayed to give me the strength to go on. I had my daughter and husband who needed me, but I just didn't want to go through it. I already had one eighteen-inch scar from the kidney and another from them opening my bladder. Each time, they took part of my bladder with the surgery.

I lost my second kidney on April 15, 2010. I woke up in ICU not knowing anything. Your kidneys maintain blood pressure, red blood cells, and many other things. My body had no idea what was happening. They couldn't get my blood pressure under control, and I almost died. I had a newly placed chest catheter for dialysis and immediately started on dialysis three times per week. You cannot live without any kidneys. They gave me twenty-two months to live at that point.

Dialysis is one scary thing to go through. There are all kinds of problems associated with dialysis. Three months after being put on dialysis, they decided that I needed a fistula put in my arm because it is dangerous to keep a chest catheter more than six months. This is a procedure where they cut your arm from the elbow to the armpit and move the deep artery out of your arm to the surface. They connect it with a vein as well. So when they put the steel dialysis needles in, one goes in the arterial side, and one goes in the venous side. This takes four months to cure before they can stick it. Once it cured, they removed the chest catheter. They hook you up, and you run for four hours in an effort to clean all your blood and put it back in. I do this three days a week. I have no way to get fluid out of my body except through dialysis. I do not consume more than twenty-four ounces of fluid a day or less.

In May of 2010, I had a severe headache for a week. I had been to the emergency room on three separate occasions that week.

On Monday, Memorial Day, I woke up and couldn't see. They took me to the hospital. The hospital released me and said that I was drug seeking. I had been on high levels of Dilaudid because of the kidney surgeries, and I had since been diagnosed with chronic fatigue syndrome, reflex sympathetic dystrophy, restless legs syndrome, neuropathy, and psuedotumor cerebri. They never checked my blood pressure and gave me an antinausea drug and sent me home.

My friend put me to bed and went downstairs to fix dinner. When she came back to check on me, I was having a seizure in the bed. They called an ambulance and returned me to the hospital forty-five minutes after I had left. They had me in ICU. They thought that my brain was bleeding in nine spots, and they did not think that I would live through the night.

My sister and friend got in touch with my primary, and because they had sent me home and almost killed me, the emergency room people were secluding my family in the back part of the hospital. My family refused for me to see the same doctor on my return.

Thank God for my family and their tenacity. They had me moved to the Mayo Clinic where I spent several weeks in ICU. I could not speak, move my arms of legs, or do anything. I would tell them ever day that I had a dream that I had died and went to the Mayo Clinic. I ended up being diagnosed with posterior reversible encephalopathy. Cape Canaveral Hospital wanted to drill holes in my brain and do a biopsy. My family refused. Once they contacted Mayo, they seemed to know what was wrong. They were working feverishly to get my blood pressure under control. Because I had lost both kidneys, my blood pressure can only be controlled with medicine and dialysis.

I was released several weeks later. I, in fact, did not live, but they revived me. I actually remember seeing a very bright white light when I died and someone with the likes of Mary as we know her motioning me away from the light. It was an experience that changed my life. I did not remember it then; it was months later that it came back and made sense. I sat down to play the piano and, to my dismay, found that I could no longer play anything but the key of C. Music that I had played for thirty years I could no longer play.

Many things had changed for me as far as intelligence, puzzle ability, working with my hands, and even walking distances. I was not able to do the things I had always done.

Several months after losing the second kidney, I developed another bladder cancer. This one had gone from low-grade low aggression to high-grade high aggression. They said that I needed to lose my entire bladder or the cancer would spread further. Little did we know, it already had. They removed my entire bladder in March of 2011. They had since been watching a spot on my lung. They went in and biopsied it, and it turned out to be neuroendocrine carcinoid. I had my right lower and middle lobe of my lung removed in May 2011. This was quite an experience for me because now I had a lung that collapsed each and every time that I bend over. All the things I took for granted were now out of my reach. It took every ounce of energy to take a shower and get dressed. I went into a very deep, dark place. It seemed like no matter what I did and how hard I prayed, I still kept getting cancer. This was my thirty-first surgery. Yes, some were minor like knees and shoulders, but the rest were pretty intensive. I have had nine bladder and ureter cancers, all ranging from transitional cell carcinoma to papillary urothelial carcinoma. I have had both kidneys and a lung removed and a total hysterectomy because of tumors and multiple other surgeries. In fact, I think I should have the record for having the least amount of organs and being still alive.

Chapter 6

Trials and Tribulations

I have had several defining moments in my life. When I was sixteen, I lived with my sister and her ex-husband. Her ex-husband got me into cocaine. I had a gram-and-a-half-cocaine habit a day. I would get up at 2:00 AM and help my sister with their paper route, go to school, and then work at Winn-Dixie at night.

One morning my father called me and told me to get into the house right away. I had a dream several nights before that something had happened to my mother, and I saw a notepad, a note, and her sitting in the bathroom. I immediately flashed to that. My second thought was my sister had told my dad that I was doing cocaine, and I was about to get blasted.

I pulled up to the house and saw my mother's car out front. I knew right away where she was. I went in the house and straight to the back to the bathroom. They were pouring coffee down her throat. She had ingested 180 muscle relaxers and gone to bed. She had woken in the morning to take a shower and passed out in the tub. She thought my brother would find her first because my dad worked nights. Fortunately, my father found her.

They rushed her to the hospital, and she was in intensive care. They said if she lived, she would be a vegetable from the brain damage. She actually lived and was not horribly brain damaged. It changed her a lot and, I think, for the better.

Mom was an opera singer and sang on Broadway when she was fifteen. She had many starring roles and had a beautiful voice. I remember playing her lines for her on the piano when I was little. I remember all the operas and the shows we got to see. My mother tried to commit suicide two other times, or so the stories go. I could never figure out why. She left a note that my father guarded. I read the note, and it said how she always loved my brother more, etc. This was a life-changing event for me. I knew she probably did love me too to some degree, but she made it pretty clear that she was not my best fan. I always felt like she didn't love me much. I made peace with her before she died, thank God.

I look back now on how much I love my daughter and can't imagine life without her. I can't fathom how someone can't love their own children. I guess in her own way, she did love me to some degree, but she actually put it in writing. This scarred me emotionally for years. I always remember thinking, *How can they not love me?* I was smart, a straight-A student, played eleven instruments, and had a profound love of life. I had survived the bone tumor at seven, the headaches, and everything else life had dished out. I finally understood that I couldn't make anyone love me.

It was at that point in my life that I decided if I ever had children that they would know they were loved to my very core being. I would not continue the cycle of corporal punishment, and I would pursue every talent they had. I realized that I was responsible for my happiness and no one else. If I didn't want to feel unloved, I didn't have to. I picked myself up by the bootstraps, as my grandfather used to say. I realized that my parents were a product of their upbringing.

Chapter 7

My Philosophy

Many times, people ask me how I do it. They ask me how I get up every morning and function. They want to know how I can keep a smile on my face. My primary-care doctor every month sees me. She asks me why I am not depressed. My answer to everyone and all these questions is that I am alive. What a gift I have been given by God to be able to still walk and talk. I have died, been dissected apart, and I am still able to walk and talk. Most people on dialysis are in wheelchairs within the first year. Dialysis destroys the nerves in your legs and hinders you, making you unable to walk.

I am so fortunate that I keep going. I have battled being on such high levels of drugs and then taking myself off them. I was up to thirty-two milligrams a day of Dilaudid, which is enough to kill a horse. I was walking, talking, and functioning like there was nothing in me. Pills scare me, and the doctors just keep giving them to me. My pain-management doctor is floored when I bring him back a prescription for pain drugs I didn't even fill. I am allergic to all pain drugs except two. I tell the doctor that I will not take them if I can't get off because it is the only one I can take. If I overtake it, then it will be useless.

I took a logic class in college, and it was at this time that many things in my life became even clearer. I had to write my beliefs and values. Values are things that we pick up from parents, educators, and those types people that we interact with every day when we are young. They form our values. I realized that what I thought was right and wrong before I cracked my head when I was thirteen was not necessarily what I now considered to be a value. Most people go through life with that same set of beliefs and values. I was fortunate and got to rethink those because I lost most memories when I cracked my head. It allowed me to look at things from the outside and evaluate whether those thoughts and opinions were justified. I think cracking my head made me a much better person. I no longer carried prejudice or disdain. I was able to think things through and make that call.

If you get nothing out of this book, know and understand that you have the power to change most any situation. You do not have to stay in bad situations. God will provide a way out for you if you ask and listen.

I think that I will eventually pursue my dream of making it to Egypt and the Holy Land. My mother was Jewish, and we were going to go to Jerusalem the year that I lost my second kidney. I have to say that other than Egypt, I have fulfilled every dream I ever had outside of writing this book. This has been a healing experience for me, and I can only hope that if you are suffering, this book will help you find peace. It is possible to beat all odds. It is possible to live without most major organs . . . just ask me.

Epilogue

My sister and I have had our ups and downs over the years as all siblings have. We sometimes agree to disagree. However, she has been a godsend to me. She has been by my side with my best friend through the most trying years. Her husband suffered from throat cancer the same time I was going through all my cancers. My niece actually became a nurse. Although we are not as close as we could be these days, I am very fortunate. You can't pick your family; they are given to you. Be thankful for whatever and whoever you have.

I met my best friend nineteen years ago. She is my daughter's godmother. Many times she drives me crazy, but I would not want her anywhere but in my life. Life gives you very few people that you can trust and call a true friend. Make sure you always hold on to them.

I thank God every day that I have a daughter that is still alive. She is twenty-three and pursuing a master's degree in geophysics at the University of Florida. She is my inspiration. She is very close to me, and I wouldn't want it any other way. I have very few close friends, but the ones I have are worth everything to me. I am supposed to die in December if the doctors are right. I don't think so.

I named the book *A Higher Calling* because I believe that God has left me here for a reason. Every time I am in the hospital, the doctors come in and tell me that there is truly no way that I should be alive. I don't look sick for the best part. I grew up in a private Christian school and knew who God was and had a very strong foundation in Christianity. I talked to God all the time. However, I never listened. He guided me like a sixth sense. I knew when I did things that were wrong and that they were bad like any other child. However, as I got older, I kept getting direction but was not listening. I believe I have learned to listen somewhat.

Over and over again it was the same message from all different people and the message was to write a book. I would be remiss to not thank the individuals responsible for me still being here medically. Great thanks to Dr. Richard Gayles, Maria, the nurses at Space Coast Pain Institute, Dr. Ziadie, Dr. Castro and Karen Tower for taking such phenomenal care of me. Thanks to Dr. Naumoff and Marilyn for finally finding the cancer. Thanks to Dr. Seth Glick for the many operations and follow-ups. Last but not least, thanks to Dr. Paul Brazis and Dr. Thiel from the Mayo. My most heartfelt wishes and thanks to these doctors and nurse practitioners as well as my family and friends. To my sister, I love you and thanks for being by my side. To my best friend, America, thanks for all you do for Kara and I. To my niece, Ashley, the nurse, you are the greatest and I love you. Thanks for always being there for all my stupid questions and needs. A special thanks to my brother in law, Mike Brace, who fought valiantly and has been an inspiration to me as well. Without all of these people, I would not be alive. In closing, my only comment is to keep the faith. Thanks for being my angels and helping where you could.

www.ingramcontent.com/pod-product-compliance
Lightning Source LLC
Chambersburg PA
CBHW061228280526
45784CB00006B/2684